Anti-Inflammatory Diet

Recipe Book 2021

Ultimate Anti-Inflammatory Diet Recipe Book
with Gorgeous Dishes for Eliminate
Inflammations Quickly!

Susie Kessler

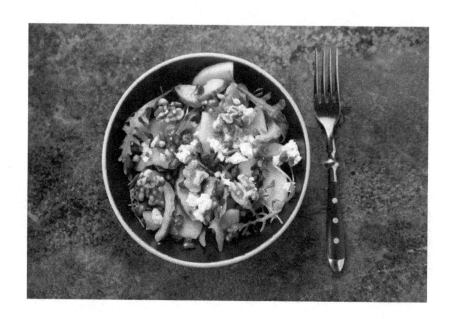

Table of Contents

INTRODUCTION 7

WINTER CHICKEN WITH VEGETABLES.................................... 13
PANCETTA & CHEESE STUFFED CHICKEN 15
CHILI CHICKEN KEBAB WITH GARLIC DRESSING 17
CHILI & LEMON MARINATED CHICKEN WINGS 19
CIPOLLINI & BELL PEPPER CHICKEN SOUVLAKI..................... 21
TARRAGON CHICKEN WITH ROASTED BALSAMIC TURNIPS 23
TOMATO & CHEESE CHICKEN CHILI 25
TURMERIC CHICKEN WINGS WITH GINGER SAUCE................. 27
FETA & BACON CHICKEN 29
CHICKEN PIE WITH BACON 31
FLYING JACOB CASSEROLE 34
BBQ CHICKEN ZUCCHINI BOATS... 36
CASHEW CHICKEN CURRY.. 38
CREAMY CHICKEN & GREENS 41
CURRY CHICKEN LETTUCE WRAPS 43
NACHO CHICKEN CASSEROLE 45
PESTO & MOZZARELLA CHICKEN CASSEROLE......................... 47
ROTISSERIE CHICKEN & CABBAGE SHREDS 49
CHICKEN QUICHE 50
CHICKEN PARMIGIANA.. 52
VODKA DUCK FILLETS.. 55
BAKED CHICKEN MEATBALLS - HABANERO & GREEN CHILI ... 57
BBQ CHICKEN LIVER AND HEARTS 59
BUFFALO BALLS... 61
TURKEY CHILI.. 63

MEAT 66

BEEF WITH CARROT & BROCCOLI.. 66
BEEF WITH MUSHROOM & BROCCOLI 68
CITRUS BEEF WITH BOK CHOY 70
BEEF WITH ZUCCHINI NOODLES 73
BEEF WITH ASPARAGUS & BELL PEPPER 75
SPICED GROUND BEEF.. 77
GROUND BEEF WITH CABBAGE... 80
GROUND BEEF WITH VEGGIES.. 82
GROUND BEEF WITH CASHEWS & VEGGIES 84
GROUND BEEF WITH GREENS & TOMATOES 86
BEEF & VEGGIES CHILI... 88

GROUND BEEF & VEGGIES CURRY 90

SPICY & CREAMY GROUND BEEF CURRY 92

CURRIED BEEF MEATBALLS 95

BEEF MEATBALLS IN TOMATO GRAVY 98

PORK WITH LEMONGRASS 101

PORK WITH OLIVES 103

PORK CHOPS WITH TOMATO SALSA 105

MUSTARD PORK MIX 107

PORK WITH CHILI ZUCCHINIS AND TOMATOES 109

PORK WITH THYME SWEET POTATOES 111

PORK WITH PEARS AND GINGER 113

PARSLEY PORK AND ARTICHOKES 115

PORK WITH MUSHROOMS AND CUCUMBERS 117

OREGANO PORK 119

CONCLUSION **121**

such, any inattention, use, or misuse of the information in question by the reader will render any resulting actions solely under their purview. There are no scenarios in which the publisher or the original author of this work can be in any fashion deemed liable for any hardship or damages that may befall them after undertaking information described herein. Additionally, the information in the following pages is intended only for informational purposes and should thus be thought of as universal. As befitting its nature, it is presented without assurance regarding its prolonged validity or interim quality. Trademarks that are mentioned are done without written consent and can in no way be considered an endorsement from the trademark holder.

Introduction

Most of the widely consumed diets incorporate anti-inflammation diet principles. In particular, the Mediterranean diet has whole grains, fish, and fats that are beneficial for the heart. Studies suggest that this diet can help lower the effects of cardiovascular system inflammation due to diet. Taking an anti-inflammatory diet is can be a complementary therapy for most conditions that are aggravated by chronic inflammation.

An anti-inflammation diet entails eating only particular kinds of food and avoiding others to lower the symptoms of chronic inflammatory diseases. It is one of the recommended measures that an individual can take to reduce or prevent inflammation induced by diet.

Expectedly, an anti-inflammatory diet involves nutrient-dense plant foods and minimizing or avoiding processed meats and foods. The goal of an anti-inflammation diet is to minimize inflammatory responses. The diet entails substituting refined foods with whole and nutrient-laden foods. Predictably, an anti-inflammation diet will contain more amounts of antioxidants that are reactive molecules in food and help reduce the number of free radicals. The free radicals are molecules in the human body that may harm cells and enhance the risk of certain diseases.

In particular, an anti-inflammation diet can help with the following diseases/conditions:

- Diabetes

Focusing exclusively on type 2 diabetes arises when the body fails to properly utilize insulin leading to higher than normal blood sugar levels. The condition of more sugar levels in the blood than normal is also known as hyperglycemia. It is also called insulin resistance. At the beginning of type 2 diabetes, the pancreas tries to make more insulin but fails to catch up with the rising blood sugar levels.

- Inflammatory bowel disease

Inflammatory bowel disease is a common gastrointestinal disorder that affects the large intestine. The symptoms of inflammatory bowel disease include abdominal pain, cramping, bloating, constipation, and diarrhea. It is a chronic condition, and it has to be managed in the long-term. Dietary measures are necessary to prevent diet-induced bloating, abdominal pain, diarrhea, and constipation. However, only a small percentage of individuals with inflammatory bowel disease will have extreme symptoms manifestation.

· Obesity

Medically, obesity refers to a complex disorder involving excessive amounts of body fat. Expectedly, obesity increases the risk of heart diseases as well as other health problems. Fortunately, modest weight loss can help halt and reverse the effects of obesity. Dietary adjustments can help address the causes of obesity, and the anti-inflammatory diet is inherently a healthy diet.

· Heart disease

Cardiovascular diseases can be triggered by diet, and diet can is used to manage several heart diseases. Food-related factors that increase the risk of heart diseases include obesity and high blood pressure. The type of fat eaten can also worsen or lesser risk of developing heart disease. In particular, cholesterol, saturated and trans fats are thought to increase heart attack rates. Most obese individuals also tend to have high-fat diets.

• Metabolic syndrome

Medically, metabolic syndrome refers to a group of factors that manifest together, leading to an increase in the risk of developing other inflammatory conditions. Some of these conditions include high blood pressure, excess body fat, especially around the waist, abnormal cholesterol, and high blood sugar levels. Having any or all of these conditions signifies that you are at a higher risk of developing a chronic condition. Most of these conditions are also associated with consuming an inflammation diet.

- Hashimoto's disease

Hashimoto's disease is an autoimmune disorder in which the body attacks its own tissues and, in particular, the thyroid organ. The result of unmanaged Hashimoto's disease is hypothyroidism implying that the body will not make adequate hormones. The thyroid gland makes hormones that control body metabolism, which includes heart rate and calories utilization. Unchecked Hashimoto's disease will also result in difficulties in swallowing when goiter manifests. Diet adjustments can be used to help manage the disease along with medications.

- Lupus

Lupus is another autoimmune disease that occurs when the body attacks its own organs and tissues. The inflammation occasioned by unmanaged lupus will affect other parts of the body. For instance, inflammation triggered by lupus will affect the heart, lungs, kidneys, and skin, including the brain and blood cells. The common symptoms of lupus are fever, fatigue, chest pain, dry eyes, and butterfly-shaped rash. Diet can be used to minimize the worsening of inflammation by adhering to the anti-inflammatory diet. The other benefit of taking an anti-inflammation diet is that it can help lower the risk of select cancers such as colorectal cancer.

Winter Chicken with Vegetables

Preparation Time: 5 minutes

Cooking Time: 30 minutes

Servings: 2

Ingredients:

- 2 tbsp. olive oil
- 2 cups whipping cream
- 1 pound chicken breasts, chopped
- 1 onion, chopped
- 1 carrot, chopped
- 2 cups chicken stock
- Salt and black pepper, to taste
- 1 bay leaf
- 1 turnip, chopped
- 1 parsnip, chopped
- 1 cup green beans, chopped
- 2 tsp fresh thyme, chopped

Directions:

1. Heat a pan at medium heat and warm the olive oil.
   Sauté the onion for 3 minutes, pour in the stock,

carrot, turnip, parsnip, chicken, and bay leaf. Place to a boil, and simmer for 20 minutes.

2. Add in the asparagus and cook for 7 minutes. Discard the bay leaf, stir in the whipping cream, adjust the seasoning, and scatter it with fresh thyme to serve.

Nutrition:

Calories 483

Fat 32.5g

Net Carbs 6.9g

Protein 33g

Pancetta & Cheese Stuffed Chicken

Preparation Time: 15 minutes

Cooking Time: 25 minutes

Servings: 2

Ingredients:

- 4 slices pancetta
- 2 tbsp. olive oil
- 2 chicken breasts
- 1 garlic clove, minced
- 1 shallot, finely chopped
- 2 tbsp. dried oregano
- 4 oz. mascarpone cheese
- 1 lemon, zested
- Salt and black pepper to taste

Directions:

1. Warm the oil in a small skillet, then sauté the garlic and shallots for 3 minutes. Stir in salt, black pepper, and lemon zest. Transfer to a bowl and let it cool. Stir in the mascarpone cheese and oregano.

2. Score a pocket in each chicken's breast, fill the holes with the cheese mixture and cover it with the

cut-out chicken. Wrap each breast with two pancetta slices and secure the ends with a toothpick.

3. Set the chicken on a greased baking sheet and cook in the oven for 20 minutes at 380 F.

Nutrition:

Calories 643

Fat 44.5g

Net Carbs 6.2g

Protein 52.8g

Chili Chicken Kebab with Garlic Dressing

Preparation Time: 7 minutes

Cooking Time: 10 minutes

Servings: 2-4

Ingredients:

- Skewers
- 2 tbsp. olive oil
- 3 tbsp. soy sauce, sugar-free
- 1 tbsp. ginger paste
- 2 tbsp. swerve brown sugar
- Chili pepper to taste
- 2 chicken breasts, cut into cubes
- Dressing
- ½ cup tahini
- 1 tbsp. parsley, chopped
- 1 garlic clove, minced
- Salt and black pepper to taste
- ¼ cup warm water

Directions:

1. To make the marinade:

2. In a small bowl, place and mix the soy sauce, ginger paste, brown sugar, chili pepper, and olive oil. Put the chicken in a zipper bag, pour the marinade over, seal, and shake for an even coat. Marinate in the fridge for 2 hours.

3. Preheat a grill to high heat. Thread the chicken on skewers and cook for 10 minutes, with three to four turnings to be golden brown. Transfer to a plate.

4. Mix the tahini, garlic, salt, parsley, and warm water in a bowl. Serve the chicken skewers topped with the tahini dressing.

Nutrition:

Calories 410

Fat 32g

Net Carbs 4.8g

Protein 23.5g

Chili & Lemon Marinated Chicken Wings

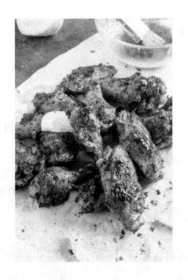

Preparation Time: 5 minutes

Cooking Time: 12 minutes

Servings: 2-4

Ingredients:

- 3 tbsp. olive oil
- 1 tsp coriander seeds
- 1 tsp xylitol
- 1 pound wings
- Juice from 1 lemon

- ½ cup fresh parsley, chopped
- 2 garlic cloves, minced
- 1 red chili pepper, chopped
- Salt and black pepper, to taste
- Lemon wedges, for serving
- ½ tsp cilantro

Directions:

1. Using a bowl, stir together lemon juice, xylitol, garlic, salt, red chili pepper, cilantro, olive oil, and black pepper. Place in the chicken wings and toss well to coat. Refrigerate for 2 hours.
2. Preheat grill over high heat. Add the chicken wings, and grill each side for 6 minutes. Serve the chicken wings with lemon wedges.

Nutrition:

Calories 223

Fat 12g

Net Carbs 5.1g

Protein 16.8g

Cipollini & Bell Pepper Chicken Souvlaki

Preparation Time: 5 minutes

Cooking Time: 12 minutes

Servings: 2-4

Ingredients:

- 2 chicken breasts, cubed
- 2 tbsp. olive oil
- 2 cloves garlic, minced
- 1 red bell pepper, cut into chunks
- 8 oz. small cipollini
- ½ cup lemon juice
- Salt and black pepper to taste
- 1 tsp rosemary leaves to garnish
- 2 to 4 lemon wedges to garnish

Directions:

1. Thread the chicken, bell pepper, and cipollini onto skewers and set aside. In a bowl, mix half of the oil, garlic, salt, black pepper, and lemon juice, and add the chicken skewers. Cover the bowl and let the

chicken marinate for at least 2 hours in the refrigerator.

2. Preheat a grill to high heat and grill the skewers for 6 minutes on each side. Remove and serve garnished with rosemary leaves and lemons wedges.

Nutrition:

Calories 363

Fat 14.2g

Net Carbs 4.2g

Protein 32.5g

Tarragon Chicken with Roasted Balsamic Turnips

Preparation Time: 10 minutes

Cooking Time: 50 minutes

Servings: 2-4

Ingredients:

- 1 pound chicken thighs
- 2 lb. turnips, cut into wedges
- 2 tbsp. olive oil
- 1 tbsp. balsamic vinegar
- 1 tbsp. tarragon
- Salt and black pepper, to taste

Directions:

1. Set the oven to 400°F then grease a baking dish with olive oil. Cook turnips in boiling water for 10 minutes, drain and set aside. Add the chicken and turnips to the baking dish.

2. Sprinkle with tarragon, black pepper, and salt. Roast for 35 minutes. Remove the baking dish, drizzle the turnip wedges with balsamic vinegar and return to the oven for another 5 minutes.

Nutrition:

Calories: 383

Fat: 26g

Net Carbs: 9.5g

Protein: 21.3g

Tomato & Cheese Chicken Chili

Preparation Time: 5 minutes

Cooking Time: 25 minutes

Servings: 2-4

Ingredients:

- 1 tbsp. butter
- 1 tbsp. olive oil
- 1 pound chicken breasts, skinless, boneless, cubed
- ½ onion, chopped
- 2 cups chicken broth
- 2 cups tomatoes, chopped
- 2 oz. tomato puree
- 1 tbsp. chili powder
- 1 tbsp. cumin
- 1 garlic clove, minced
- 1 habanero pepper, minced
- ½ cup mozzarella cheese, shredded
- Salt and black pepper to taste

Directions:

1. Season the chicken using salt and pepper. Set a large pan at medium heat and add the chicken;

cover it with water, and bring it to a boil. Cook until no longer pink, for 10 minutes.

2. Transfer the chicken to a flat surface to shred with forks. In a pot, pour in the butter and olive oil and set over medium heat. Sauté onion and garlic until transparent for 5 minutes.

3. Stir in the chicken, tomatoes, cumin, habanero pepper, tomato puree, broth, and chili powder. Adjust the seasoning and let the mixture boil.

4. Reduce heat to simmer for about 10 minutes. Top with shredded cheese to serve.

Nutrition:

Calories: 322

Fat: 16.6g

Net Carbs: 6.2g

Protein: 29g

Turmeric Chicken Wings with Ginger Sauce

Preparation Time: 5 minutes

Cooking Time: 20 minutes

Servings: 2-4

Ingredients:

- 2 tbsp. olive oil
- 1 pound chicken wings, cut in half
- 1 tbsp. turmeric
- 1 tbsp. cumin
- 3 tbsp. fresh ginger, grated
- Salt and black pepper, to taste
- Juice of ½ lime
- 1 cup thyme leaves
- ¾ cup cilantro, chopped
- 1 tbsp. water
- 1 jalapeño pepper

Directions:

1. In a bowl, stir together 1 tbsp. ginger, cumin, and salt, half of the olive oil, black pepper, turmeric,

and cilantro. Place in the chicken wings pieces, toss to coat, and refrigerate for 20 minutes.

2. Heat the grill to high heat. Remove the wings from the marinade, drain, and grill for 20 minutes, turning from time to time, then set aside.

3. Using a blender, combine thyme, remaining ginger, salt, jalapeno pepper, black pepper, lime juice, the remaining olive oil, and water, and blend well.

Serve the chicken wings topped with the sauce.

Nutrition:
Calories 253

Fat 16.1g

Net Carbs 4.1g

Protein 21.7g

Feta & Bacon Chicken

Preparation Time: 20 minutes

Cooking Time: 10minutes

Servings: 2-4

Ingredients:

- 4 oz. bacon, chopped
- 1 pound chicken breasts
- 3 green onions, chopped
- 2 tbsp. coconut oil
- 4 oz. feta cheese, crumbled
- 1 tbsp. parsley

Directions:

1. Place a pan over medium heat and coat with cooking spray. Add in the bacon and cook until crispy. Remove to paper towels, drain the grease and crumble.

2. To the same pan, add in the oil and cook the chicken breasts for 4-5 minutes, then flip to the other side; cook for an additional 4-5 minutes. Place the chicken breasts to a baking dish. Place the green onions, set in the oven, turn on the broiler,

and cook for 5 minutes at high temperature. Remove to serving plates and serve topped with bacon, feta cheese, and parsley.

Nutrition:

Calories 459

Fat 35g

Net Carbs 3.1g

Protein 31.5g

Chicken Pie with Bacon

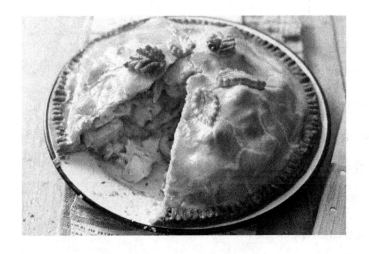

Preparation Time: 20 minutes

Cooking Time: 35 minutes

Servings: 24

Ingredients:

- 3 tbsp. butter
- 1 onion, chopped
- 4 oz. bacon, sliced
- 1 carrot, chopped
- 3 garlic cloves, minced
- Salt and black pepper, to taste
- ¾ cup crème fraîche

- ½ cup chicken stock

- 1 pound chicken breasts, cubed

- 2 tbsp. yellow mustard

- ¾ cup cheddar cheese, shredded

- Dough

- 1 egg

- ¾ cup almond flour

- 3 tbsp. cream cheese

- 1 ½ cups mozzarella cheese, shredded

- 1 tsp onion powder

- 1 tsp garlic powder

- Salt and black pepper, to taste

Directions:

1. Sauté the onion, garlic, black pepper, bacon, and carrot in melted butter for 5 minutes. Add in the chicken and cook for 3 minutes. Stir in the crème fraîche, salt, mustard, black pepper, and stock, and cook for 7 minutes. Add in the cheddar cheese and set aside.

2. In a bowl, combine the mozzarella cheese with the cream cheese and heat in a microwave for 1 minute. Stir in the garlic powder, salt, flour, black pepper,

onion powder, and egg. Knead the dough well, split into 4 pieces, and flatten each into a circle.

3. Set the chicken mixture into 4 ramekins, top each with a dough circle, and cook in the oven at 370 F for 25 minutes.

Nutrition:
Calories 563

Fat 44.6g

Net Carbs 7.7g

Protein 36g

Flying Jacob Casserole

Preparation Time: 15 minutes

Cooking Time: 20-25 minutes

Servings: 6

Ingredients:

- 1 pc Grilled Chicken
- 2 tbsp. Butter
- 225 g Diced bacon
- 250 g Mushrooms
- 475 ml Cream
- 125 ml hot chili sauce
- 1 tsp. Seasoning curry
- Salt and black pepper to taste
- 125 g Peanuts
- Salad
- 175 g Spinach
- 2 pcs Tomato

Directions:

1. Preheat the oven to 400 ° F.
2. Chop the mushrooms into small pieces then fry in oil with bacon. Salt and pepper to taste.

3. Separate the chicken meat from the bones and chop it into small pieces.

4. Put these pieces of chicken in a mold for baking, oiled. Add mushrooms and bacon.

5. Beat the cream until soft peaks. Put chili sauce, curry, and salt and pepper to taste.

6. Pour the chicken into the resulting mixture.

7. Bake in the oven for at least 20-25 minutes until the dish will get a pleasant golden color. Sprinkle toasted and chopped nuts on top. Serve with salad.

Nutrition:

Carbohydrates: 11 g

Fats: 80 g

Proteins: 40 g

Calories: 912

BBQ Chicken Zucchini Boats

Preparation Time: 10 minutes

Cooking Time: 15-20 minutes

Servings: 4

Ingredients:

- 3 Zucchini halved
- 1 lb. cooked Chicken breast
- .5 cup BBQ sauce
- .33 cup Shredded Mexican cheese
- 1 Avocado, sliced
- .5 cup Halved cherry tomatoes
- .25 cup Diced green onions
- 3 tbsp. Keto-friendly ranch dressing
- Also Needed: 9x13 casserole dish

Directions:

1. Set the oven to reach 350° Fahrenheit.

2. Using a knife, cut the zucchini in half. Discard the seeds. Make the boat by carving out of the center. Place the zucchini flesh side up into the casserole dish.

3. Discard and cut the skin and bones from the chicken. Shred and add the chicken in with the barbeque sauce. Toss to coat all the chicken fully.

4. Fill the zucchini boats with the mixture using about .25 to .33 cup each.

5. Sprinkle with Mexican cheese on top.

6. Bake for approximately 15 minutes. (If you would like it tenderer; bake for an additional 5 to 10 minutes to reach the desired tenderness.)

7. Remove from the oven. Top it off with avocado, green onion, tomatoes, and a drizzle of dressing. Serve.

Nutrition:

Calories: 212

Net Carbs: 9 g

Total Fat Content: 11 g

Protein: 19 g

Cashew Chicken Curry

Preparation Time: 15 minutes

Cooking Time: 25 minutes

Servings: 4

Ingredients:

- 1 cups Cauliflower

- 2 large fresh tomatoes

- 1 medium Red onion

- 2 cups Cucumber

- 2 tbsp. Coconut oil

- 1 tbsp. & .5 tsp. Yellow curry powder - divided

- Sea salt & Black pepper (as desired)

- .66 cup Roasted - salted cashews (

- 1.lb Breasts of chicken, 4 small

- 1 large Egg white

- For the Garnish:

- Freshly chopped fresh mint

- Minced fresh cilantro

- Also Needed: Food processor & Rimmed baking sheet

Directions:

1. Chop the cauliflower into florets and quarter the tomatoes. Roughly chop the onion and thinly slice the cucumber into halves. Take off the skin and bones from the chicken.

2. Heat the oven to 425° Fahrenheit.

3. Toss the quartered tomatoes, cauliflower florets, and onion into a mixing container. Melt the coconut oil and sprinkle using 1.5 teaspoons of curry powder. Mix until well.

4. Prepare on a baking sheet in one layer. Dust with pepper and salt to your liking. Add the rest of the curry powder and cashews into a food processor. Pulse leaving a few chunks for texture.

5. Pat to remove the moisture from the chicken breasts using a paper towel.

6. Put the egg white and cashews into two shallow plates.

7. Dredge the chicken through the egg white. Shake off any excess, and press into the cashews.

8. Flip and lightly press the other side into the cashews.

9. Put the chicken breast onto a small cooling rack that fits on your sheet pan (one with legs is preferred, so it sits over the veggies).

10. Continue the process with the remaining chicken. Place the cooling rack over a sheet pan (over the top of the veggies).

11. Bake the chicken to reach an internal temperature of 165° Fahrenheit (14-15 min.). Once it's done, toss the fresh cucumbers onto the pan. Garnish with mint and cilantro.

Nutrition:

Calories: 364

Net Carbs: 14 g

Total Fat Content: 18 g

Protein: 34 g

Creamy Chicken & Greens

Preparation Time: 10 minutes

Cooking Time: 20 minutes

Servings: 4

Ingredients:

- 1 lb. Chicken thighs – skins on
- 1 cup. Chicken stock
- 1 cup. Cream
- 2 tbsp. Coconut oil
- 1 tsp. Italian herbs
- 2 cups Dark leafy greens
- Pepper & Salt (your preference)
- 2 tbsp. Coconut flour
- 2 tbsp. Melted butter

Directions:

1. On the stovetop, add oil in a skillet using the med-high temperature setting.

2. Remove the bones from the chicken and dust using salt and pepper. Fry the chicken until done.

3. Make the sauce by adding the butter to a saucepan. Whisk in the flour to form a thick paste. Slowly, whisk in the cream. Once it boils, mix in the herbs.

4. Transfer the chicken to the counter and add the stock.

5. Deglaze the pan, and whisk the cream sauce. Toss in the greens until thoroughly coated with the sauce.

6. Arrange the thighs on the greens, warm up, and serve.

Nutrition:

Calories: 446

Net Carbs: 3 g

Total Fat Content: 38 g

Protein: 18 g

Curry Chicken Lettuce Wraps

Preparation Time: 15 minutes

Cooking Time: 10 minutes

Servings: 5

Ingredients:

- 2 Minced garlic cloves
- .25 cups Minced onion
- 1 lb. Chicken thighs – skinless & boneless
- 2 tbsp. Ghee
- 1 tsp. Black pepper
- 2 tsp. Curry powder
- 1.5 tsp. Salt
- 1 cup Riced cauliflower
- 5-6 Lettuce leaves
- Keto-friendly sour cream (as desired - count the carbs)

Directions:

1. Mince the garlic and onions. Set aside for now.
2. Pull out the bones and skin from the chicken and dice into one-inch pieces.

3. On the stovetop, add 2 tbsp. of ghee to a skillet and melt. Toss in the onion and sauté until browned. Fold in the chicken and sprinkle with the garlic, pepper, and salt.

4. Cook for eight minutes. Stir in the remainder of the ghee, riced cauliflower, and curry. Stir until well mixed.

5. Prepare the lettuce leaves and add the mixture.

6. Serve with a dollop of cream.

Nutrition:

Calories: 554

Net Carbs: 7 g

Total Fat Content: 36 g

Protein: 50 g

Nacho Chicken Casserole

Preparation Time: 15 minutes

Cooking Time: 25 minutes

Servings: 6

Ingredients:

- 1 medium Jalapeño pepper
- 1.75lb. Chicken thighs
- Pepper and salt (to taste)
- 2 tbsp. Olive oil
- 1.5tsp. Chili seasoning
- 4 oz. Cheddar cheese
- 4 oz. Cream cheese
- 3 tbsp. Parmesan cheese
- 1 cup Green chilies and tomatoes
- .25 cup Sour cream
- 1 pkg. Frozen cauliflower
- Also Needed: Immersion blender

Directions:

1. Warm the oven to reach 375° Fahrenheit.
2. Slice the jalapeño into pieces and set aside.

3. Cutaway the skin and bones from the chicken. Chop it and sprinkle using the pepper and salt. Prepare in a skillet using a portion of olive oil on the med-high temperature setting until browned.

4. Mix in the sour cream, cream cheese, and ¾ of the cheddar cheese. Stir until melted and combined well. Place in the tomatoes and chilies. Stir then put it all to a baking dish.

5. Cook the cauliflower in the microwave. Blend in the rest of the cheese with the immersion blender until it resembles mashed potatoes. Season as desired.

6. Spread the cauliflower concoction over the casserole and sprinkle with the peppers. Bake approximately 15 to 20 minutes.

Nutrition:

Calories: 426

Net Carbs: 4.3 g

Total Fat Content: 32.2 g

Protein: 31 g

Pesto & Mozzarella Chicken Casserole

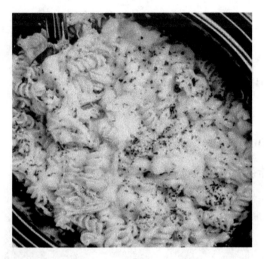

Preparation Time: 10 minutes

Cooking Time: 25-30 minutes

Servings: 8

Ingredients:

- Cooking oil (as needed)
- 2 lb. Grilled & cubed chicken breasts
- 8 oz. Cubed mozzarella
- 8 oz. Cream cheese
- 8 oz. Shredded mozzarella
- .25 cup Pesto
- .25 to .5 cup Heavy cream

Directions:

1. Warm the oven to 400° Fahrenheit. Spritz a casserole dish with a spritz of cooking oil spray.

2. Combine the pesto, heavy cream, and softened cream cheese.

3. Add the chicken and cubed mozzarella into the greased dish.

4. Sprinkle the chicken using the shredded mozzarella. Bake for 25-30 minutes.

Nutrition:

Calories: 451

Net Carbs: 3 g

Total Fat Content: 30 g

Protein: 38 g

Rotisserie Chicken & Cabbage Shreds

Preparation Time: 10 minutes

Cooking Time: 0 minutes

Servings: 2

Ingredients:

- .5 of 1 Red onion
- 7 oz. Fresh green cabbage
- 1 lb. Precooked rotisserie chicken
- .5 cup Keto-friendly mayo
- 1 tbsp. Olive oil
- Pepper & Salt

Direction:

1. Use a sharp kitchen knife to shred the cabbage and slice the onion into thin slices.
2. Place the chicken on a platter, add the mayo, and a drizzle of oil. Dust using salt and pepper. Serve.

Nutrition:

Calories: 423

Net Carbs: 6 g

Total Fat Content: 35 g

Protein: 17 g

Chicken Quiche

Preparation Time: 15 minutes

Cooking Time: 50 minutes

Servings: 6

Ingredients:

- 16 oz. almond flour
- 7 medium eggs
- Salt and ground black pepper to taste
- 2 tbsp. coconut oil
- 1 lb. ground chicken
- 2 small zucchini, grated
- 1 tsp dried oregano
- 1 tsp fennel seeds
- ½ cup heavy cream

Directions:

1. Place almond flour, 1 egg, salt, and coconut oil in blender or food processor and blend.
2. Grease pie pan and pour the dough in it. Press well on the bottom.
3. Preheat pan on medium heat and toss ground chicken, cook for 2 minutes, set aside.

4. In a medium bowl, whisk together 6 eggs, zucchini, oregano, salt, pepper, fennel seeds, and heavy cream.

5. Add chicken to egg mixture and stir well.

6. Preheat oven to 350 F.

7. Pour egg mixture into pie pan and place in oven. Cook for 40 minutes.

8. Let it cool and slice. Serve.

Nutrition:

Calories

295

Carbs 3.95g

Fat 24g

Protein 19g

Chicken Parmigiana

Preparation Time: 15 minutes

Cooking Time: 26 minutes

Servings: 4

Ingredients:

- 1 large organic egg, beaten
- ½ cup of superfine blanched almond flour
- ¼ cup Parmesan cheese, grated
- ½ teaspoon dried parsley
- ½ teaspoon paprika
- ½ teaspoon garlic powder
- Salt and ground black pepper, as required
- 4 -6-ounces grass-fed skinless, boneless chicken breasts, pounded into a ½-inch thickness
- ¼ cup olive oil
- 1½ cups marinara sauce
- 4 ounces mozzarella cheese, thinly sliced
- 2 tablespoons fresh parsley, chopped

Directions:

1. Preheat the oven to 375 degrees F.
2. Add the beaten egg into a shallow dish.

3. Place the almond flour, Parmesan, parsley, spices, salt, and black pepper in another shallow dish and mix well.

4. Dip each chicken breast into the beaten egg and then coat with the flour mixture.

5. Heat the oil in a deep skillet over medium-high heat and fry the chicken breasts for about 3 minutes per side.

6. Using a slotted spoon, moved the chicken breasts onto a paper towel-lined plate to drain.

7. At the bottom of a casserole, put about ½ cup of marinara sauce and spread evenly.

8. Arrange the chicken breasts over marinara sauce in a single layer.

9. Top with the remaining marinara sauce, followed by mozzarella cheese slices.

10. Bake for about at least 20 minutes or until done completely.

11. Take off from the oven and serve hot with the garnishing of fresh parsley.

Nutrition:

Calories: 542

Net Carbs: 5.7g

Carbohydrate: 9g

Fiber: 3.3g

Protein: 54.2g

Fat: 33.2g

Sugar: 3.8g

Sodium: 609mg

Vodka Duck Fillets

Preparation Time: 5 minutes

Cooking Time: 15 minutes

Servings: 4

Ingredients:

- 1 tablespoon lard, room temperature
- 4 duck fillets
- 4 green onions, chopped
- Salt and cayenne pepper, to taste
- 1 teaspoon mixed peppercorns
- 1 ½ cups turkey stock
- 3 tablespoons Worcestershire sauce
- 2 ounces vodka
- 1/2 teaspoon ground bay leaf
- 1/2 cup sour cream

Directions:

1. Melt the lard in a skillet that is preheated over medium-high heat. Sear the duck fillets, turning once, for 4 to 6 minutes.

2. Now, add the remaining ingredients, except for the sour cream, to the skillet. Cook, partially covered, for a further 7 minutes.

3. Serve warm, garnished with sour cream. Bon appétit!

Nutrition:

351 Calories

24.7g Fat

6.6g Carbs

22.1g Protein

Baked Chicken Meatballs - Habanero & Green Chili

Preparation Time: 10 minutes

Cooking Time: 25 minutes

Servings: 15

Ingredients:

- 1 pound ground chicken
- 1 poblano pepper
- 1 habanero pepper
- 1 jalapeno pepper
- 1/2 cup cilantro
- 1 tbsp. vinegar
- 1 tbsp. olive oil
- salt to taste

Directions:

1. Preheat broiler to 400 degrees Fahrenheit.
2. In an enormous blending bowl, join chicken, minced peppers, cilantro, salt, and vinegar with your hands. Structure 1-inch meatballs with the blend

3. Coat every meatball with olive oil, at that point, place on a rimmed heating sheet or meal dish.

4. Heat for 25 minutes

Nutrition:

Calories 54

Fat 3g

Carbs 5g

Protein 5g

BBQ Chicken Liver and Hearts

Preparation Time: 15 minutes

Cooking Time: 20 minutes

Servings: 4

Ingredients:

- 1 lb. chicken hearts
- 1 lb. chicken livers
- sea salt
- black pepper
- bamboo skewers

Directions:

1. The liver and hearts defrost and bring to room temperature.

2. The heart's extreme top parts can be evacuated with a sharp blade.

3. Meanwhile, set up the BBQ - we utilize just charcoals; however, you can utilize gas, and bring to prescription/high warmth.

4. Presently string the hearts on the sticks, 5 to 7 each, contingent upon their size.

5. After cleaning the livers, focusing not to break or smash them, lay level on an adaptable barbecuing bushel

6. Season both liver and hearts with ocean salt and naturally ground dark pepper.

7. The livers will generally stick on the barbecue and effectively break separated currently set on the flame broil and cook until the ideal doneness is come to.

Nutrition:

Calories 361

Fat 28g

Carbs 4.5g

Protein 23g

Buffalo Balls

Preparation Time: 10 minutes

Cooking Time: 40 minutes

Servings: 18

Ingredients:

- For the Meatballs:
- 1lb ground chicken or turkey
- 1/4 cup almond flour
- 2 oz. cream cheese softened
- 1 egg
- 2 tbsp. chopped celery
- 3 tbsp. crumbled blue cheese
- 1/4 tsp black pepper
- For the Sauce:
- 1/2 stick (4 oz.) unsalted butter
- 1/2 cup Frank's Red Hot

Directions:

1. In a medium bowl, put all the meatballs ingredients then mix. Form into about 1 inch balls.

2. Set it on a greased cookie sheet (with sides) and bake at 350°F for at least 10 minutes.

3. To make the sauce: put the Frank's and butter in a small saucepan on medium heat, or place in a microwave-safe bowl for 2 minutes on high.

4. After 10 minutes, remove balls from the oven and dunk carefully in the buffalo sauce.

5. Return onto the cookie sheet and bake for another 12 minutes. If you have a leftover sauce, you could pour it over the meatballs and bake for another 3 to 4 minutes if you want them saucy.

Nutrition:

Calories: 331

Fat: 28g

Carbs: 2g

Protein: 17g

Turkey Chili

Preparation Time: 5 minutes

Cooking Time: 30 minutes

Servings: 2

Ingredients:

- 1 ounce jalapeno pepper
- 1 ounce red bell pepper (or other colors)
- 3 ounces zucchini
- 1 ½ tablespoon olive oil
- 5 ounces ground turkey
- 1 cup water or as needed
- 1 ½ ounces cauliflower rice
- 1 ½ tablespoons sour cream
- 4 tablespoons shredded cheddar cheese
- ¼ teaspoon pepper
- 1 teaspoon paprika
- 1/3 teaspoon onion powder or garlic powder (optional)
- ¼ teaspoon ground cumin (optional)
- Salt to taste

Directions:

1. Chop the red bell pepper, jalapeno pepper, and zucchini into smaller, bite-sized pieces. Feel free to slice jalapeno pepper into larger pieces if you want to avoid them and control the spiciness in your mouth later on.

2. Take a large stewing pot, add the olive oil, and put it on medium heat. Put the ground turkey and cook it until it becomes brown. Use a spatula to break it up.

3. Mix bell pepper, jalapeno, and zucchini with turkey. Put a cover on your pot and let your mixture cook on a low heat for approximately 5 minutes or until you see that vegetables became a little bit softer.

4. Season everything and add water. Stir the chili.

5. Cover your pot once again and bring your mixture to a simmer. Continue to stir it for about 10 more minutes.

6. Add the cauliflower rice. Remove the cover and keep cooking at the low heat.

7. Fill approximately ½ of a cup with the liquid you remove from the pot. Place it into a clean bowl and mix it with the sour cream.

8. Bring the thickened liquid back to the pot. Stir your ingredients once again and let your chili simmer for 5 more minutes for it to thicken a little bit more.

9. While serving this meal, fill 2 bowls and top each of those with 2 tablespoons of cheddar cheese.

Nutrition:

Calories: 378

Total Carbs: 6,3g

Fiber: 2g

Net Carbs: 4,3g

Fat: 30g

Protein: 23g

Meat

Beef with Carrot & Broccoli

Preparation Time: 15 minutes

Cooking Time: 14 minutes

Servings: 4

Ingredients:

- 2 tbsp. coconut oil, divided
- 2 medium garlic cloves, minced
- 1 lb. beef sirloin steak, sliced into thin strips
- Salt, to taste
- ¼ cup chicken broth
- 2 tsp. fresh ginger, grated
- 1 tbsp. Ground flax seeds
- ½ tsp. Red pepper flakes, crushed
- ¼ tsp. freshly ground black pepper
- 1 large carrot, peeled and sliced thinly
- 2 cups broccoli florets
- 1 medium scallion, sliced thinly

Directions:

1. In a skillet, warm 1 tbsp. of oil on medium-high heat.
2. Put garlic and sauté approximately 1 minute.
3. Add beef and salt and cook for at least 4-5 minutes or till browned.
4. Using a slotted spoon, transfer the beef in a bowl.
5. Take off the liquid from the skillet.
6. In a bowl, put together broth, ginger, flax seeds, red pepper flakes, and black pepper then mix.
7. In the same skillet, warm remaining oil on medium heat.
8. Put the carrot, broccoli, and ginger mixture then cook for at least 3-4 minutes or till desired doneness.
9. Mix in beef and scallion then cook for around 3-4 minutes.

Nutrition:

Calories: 412

Fat: 13g

Carbohydrates: 28g

Fiber: 9g

Protein: 35g

Beef with Mushroom & Broccoli

Preparation Time: 15 minutes

Cooking Time: 12 minutes

Servings: 4

Ingredients:

- For Beef Marinade:
- 1 garlic clove, minced
- 1 (2-inch piece fresh ginger, minced
- Salt, to taste
- Freshly ground black pepper, to taste
- 3 tbsp. white wine vinegar
- ¾ cup beef broth
- 1 lb. flank steak, trimmed and sliced into thin strips
- For Vegetables:
- 2 tbsp. coconut oil, divided
- 2 minced garlic cloves
- 3 cups broccoli rabe, chopped
- 4 oz. shiitake mushrooms halved
- 8 oz. cremini mushrooms, sliced

Directions:

1. For marinade in a bowl, put together all ingredients except beef then mix.

2. Add beef and coat with marinade.

3. Bring in the fridge to marinate for at least 15 minutes.

4. In the skillet, warm oil on medium-high heat.

5. Take off beef from the bowl, reserving the marinade.

6. Put beef and garlic and cook for about 3-4 minutes or till browned.

7. Using a slotted spoon, transfer the beef in a bowl.

8. In the same skillet, put the reserved marinade, broccoli, and mushrooms and cook for at least 3-4 minutes.

9. Stir in beef and cook for at least 3-4 minutes.

Nutrition:

Calories: 417

Fat: 10g

Carbohydrates: 23g

Fiber: 11g

Protein: 33g

Citrus Beef with Bok Choy

Preparation Time: 15 minutes

Cooking Time: 11 minutes

Servings: 4

Ingredients:

- For Marinade:
- 2 minced garlic cloves
- 1 (1-inch piece fresh ginger, grated
- 1/3 cup fresh orange juice
- ½ cup coconut aminos
- 2 tsp. fish sauce
- 2 tsp. Sriracha
- 1¼ lb. sirloin steak, sliced thinly

For Veggies:

1. 2 tbsp. coconut oil, divided
2. 3-4 wide strips of fresh orange zest
3. 1 jalapeño pepper, sliced thinly
4. ½ pound string beans stemmed and halved crosswise
5. 1 tbsp. arrowroot powder
6. ½ pound Bok choy, chopped

7. 2 tsp. sesame seeds

Directions:

- For marinade in a big bowl, put together garlic, ginger, orange juice, coconut aminos, fish sauce, and Sriracha then mix.

- Put the beef and coat with marinade.

- Place in the fridge to marinate for around a couple of hours.

- In a skillet, warm oil on medium-high heat.

- Add orange zest and sauté approximately 2 minutes.

- Take off the beef from a bowl, reserving the marinade.

- In the skillet, add beef and increase the heat to high.

- Stir fry for at least 2-3 minutes or till browned.

- With a slotted spoon, transfer the beef and orange strips right into a bowl.

- With a paper towel, wipe out the skillet.

- In a similar skillet, heat remaining oil on medium-high heat.

- Add jalapeño pepper and string beans and stir fry for about 3-4 minutes.
- Meanwhile, add arrowroot powder in reserved marinade and stir to mix.
- In the skillet, add marinade mixture, beef, and Bok choy and cook for about 1-2 minutes.
- Serve hot with garnishing of sesame seeds.

Nutrition:

Calories: 398

Fat: 11g

Carbohydrates: 20g

Fiber: 6g

Protein: 34g

Beef with Zucchini Noodles

Preparation Time: 15 minutes

Cooking Time: 9 minutes

Servings: 4

Ingredients:

1. 1 teaspoon fresh ginger, grated
2. 2 medium garlic cloves, minced
3. ¼ cup coconut aminos
4. 2 tablespoons fresh lime juice
5. 1½ pound NY strip steak, trimmed and sliced thinly
6. 2 medium zucchinis, spiralizer with Blade C
7. Salt, to taste
8. 3 tablespoons essential olive oil
9. 2 medium scallions, sliced
10. 1 teaspoon red pepper flakes, crushed
11. 2 tablespoons fresh cilantro, chopped

Directions:

- In a big bowl, mix together ginger, garlic, coconut aminos, and lime juice.
- Add beef and coat with marinade generously.

- Refrigerate to marinate for approximately 10 minutes.

- Place zucchini noodles over a large paper towel and sprinkle with salt.

- Keep aside for around 10 minutes.

- In a big skillet, heat oil on medium-high heat.

- Add scallion and red pepper flakes and sauté for about 1 minute.

- Add beef with marinade and stir fry for around 3-4 minutes or till browned.

- Add zucchini and cook for approximately 3-4 minutes.

- Serve hot with all the topping of cilantro.

Nutrition:

Calories: 434

Fat: 17g

Carbohydrates: 23g

Fiber: 12g

Protein: 29g

Beef with Asparagus & Bell Pepper

Preparation Time: 15 minutes

Cooking Time: 13 minutes

Servings: 4-5

Ingredients:

1. 4 garlic cloves, minced
2. 3 tablespoons coconut aminos
3. 1/8 teaspoon red pepper flakes, crushed
4. 1/8 teaspoon ground ginger
5. Freshly ground black pepper, to taste
6. 1 bunch asparagus, trimmed and halved
7. 2 tablespoons olive oil, divided
8. 1-pound flank steak, trimmed and sliced thinly
9. 1 red bell pepper, seeded and sliced
10. 3 tablespoons water
11. 2 teaspoons arrowroot powder

Directions:

- In a bowl, mix together garlic, coconut aminos, red pepper flakes, crushed, ground ginger, and black pepper. Keep aside.
- In a pan of boiling water, cook asparagus for about 2 minutes.

- Drain and rinse under cold water.
- In a substantial skillet, heat 1 tablespoon of oil on medium-high heat.
- Add beef and stir fry for around 3-4 minutes.
- With a slotted spoon, transfer the beef in a bowl.
- In a similar skillet, heat remaining oil on medium heat.
- Add asparagus and bell pepper and stir fry for approximately 2-3 minutes.
- Meanwhile, in the bowl, mix together water and arrowroot powder.
- Stir in beef, garlic mixture, and arrowroot mixture, and cook for around 3-4 minutes or till desired thickness.

Nutrition:

Calories: 399

Fat: 17g

Carbohydrates: 27g

Fiber: 8g

Protein: 35g

Spiced Ground Beef

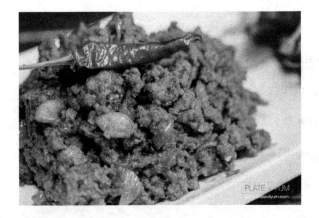

Preparation Time: 10 minutes

Cooking Time: 22 minutes

Servings: 5

Ingredients:

1. 2 tablespoons coconut oil

2. 2 whole cloves

3. 2 whole cardamoms

4. 1 (2-inch piece cinnamon stick

5. 2 bay leaves

6. 1 teaspoon cumin seeds

7. 2 onions, chopped

8. Salt, to taste

9. ½ tablespoon garlic paste

10. ½ tablespoon fresh ginger paste

11. 1-pound lean ground beef

12. 1½ teaspoons fennel seeds powder

13. 1 teaspoon ground cumin

14. 1½ teaspoons red chili powder

15. 1/8 teaspoon ground turmeric

16. Freshly ground black pepper, to taste

17. 1 cup coconut milk

18. ¼ cup water

19. ¼ cup fresh cilantro, chopped

Directions:

- In a sizable pan, heat oil on medium heat.

- Add cloves, cardamoms, cinnamon stick, bay leaves, and cumin seeds and sauté for about 20-a few seconds.

- Add onion and 2 pinches of salt and sauté for about 3-4 minutes.

- Add garlic-ginger paste and sauté for about 2 minutes.

- Add beef and cook for about 4-5 minutes, entering pieces using the spoon.

- Cover and cook approximately 5 minutes.

- Stir in spices and cook, stirring for approximately 2-2½ minutes.

- Stir in coconut milk and water and cook for about 7-8 minutes.

- Season with salt and take away from heat.

- Serve hot using the garnishing of cilantro.

Nutrition:
Calories: 444

Fat: 15g

Carbohydrates: 29g

Fiber: 11g

Protein: 39g

Ground Beef with Cabbage

Preparation Time: 10 minutes

Cooking Time: 15 minutes

Servings: 6

Ingredients:

1. 1 tbsp. olive oil
2. 1 onion, sliced thinly
3. 2 teaspoons fresh ginger, minced
4. 4 garlic cloves, minced
5. 1-pound lean ground beef
6. 1½ tablespoons fish sauce
7. 2 tablespoons fresh lime juice
8. 1 small head purple cabbage, shredded
9. 2 tablespoons peanut butter
10. ½ cup fresh cilantro, chopped

Directions:

- In a huge skillet, warm oil on medium heat.
- Add onion, ginger, and garlic and sauté for about 4-5 minutes.
- Add beef and cook for approximately 7-8 minutes, getting into pieces using the spoon.

- Drain off the extra liquid in the skillet.
- Stir in fish sauce and lime juice and cook for approximately 1 minute.
- Add cabbage and cook approximately 4-5 minutes or till desired doneness.
- Stir in peanut butter and cilantro and cook for about 1 minute.
- Serve hot.

Nutrition:

Calories: 402

Fat: 13g

Carbohydrates: 21g

Fiber: 10g

Protein: 33g

Ground Beef with Veggies

Preparation Time: 15 minutes

Cooking Time: 20 minutes

Servings: 2-4

Ingredients:

1. 1-2 tablespoons coconut oil
2. 1 red onion, sliced
3. 2 red jalapeño peppers, seeded and sliced
4. 2 minced garlic cloves
5. 1-pound lean ground beef
6. 1 small head broccoli, chopped
7. ½ of head cauliflower, chopped
8. 3 carrots, peeled and sliced
9. 3 celery ribs, sliced
10. Chopped fresh thyme, to taste
11. Dried sage, to taste
12. Ground turmeric, to taste
13. Salt, to taste
14. Freshly ground black pepper, to taste

Directions:

- In a huge skillet, melt coconut oil on medium heat.

- Add onion, jalapeño peppers and garlic and sauté for about 5 minutes.
- Add beef and cook for around 4-5 minutes, entering pieces using the spoon.
- Add remaining ingredients and cook, occasionally stirring for about 8-10 min.
- Serve hot.

Nutrition:
Calories: 453

Fat: 17g

Carbohydrates: 26g

Fiber: 8g,

Protein: 35g

Ground Beef with Cashews & Veggies

Preparation Time: 15 minutes

Cooking Time: 15 minutes

Servings: 4

Ingredients:

1. 1½ pound lean ground beef
2. 1 tablespoon garlic, minced
3. 2 tablespoons fresh ginger, minced
4. ¼ cup coconut aminos
5. Salt, to taste
6. Freshly ground black pepper, to taste
7. 1 medium onion, sliced
8. 1 can water chestnuts, drained and sliced
9. 1 large green bell pepper, sliced
10. ½ cup raw cashews, toasted

Directions:

- Heat a nonstick skillet on medium-high heat.
- Add beef and cook for about 6-8 minutes, breaking into pieces with all the spoon.
- Add garlic, ginger, coconut aminos, salt, and black pepper and cook approximately 2 minutes.

- Put the vegetables and cook approximately 5 minutes or till desired doneness.
- Stir in cashews and immediately remove from heat.
- Serve hot.

Nutrition:

Calories: 452

Fat: 20g

Carbohydrates: 26g

Fiber: 9g

Protein: 36g

Ground Beef with Greens & Tomatoes

Preparation Time: 15 minutes

Cooking Time: 15 minutes

Servings: 4

Ingredients:

1. 1 tbsp. organic olive oil

2. ½ of white onion, chopped

3. 2 garlic cloves, chopped finely

4. 1 jalapeño pepper, chopped finely

5. 1-pound lean ground beef

6. 1 teaspoon ground coriander

7. 1 teaspoon ground cumin

8. ½ teaspoon ground turmeric

9. ½ teaspoon ground ginger

10. ½ teaspoon ground cinnamon

11. ½ teaspoon ground fennel seeds

12. Salt, to taste

13. Freshly ground black pepper, to taste

14. 8 fresh cherry tomatoes, quartered

15. 8 collard greens leaves, stemmed and chopped

16. 1 teaspoon fresh lemon juice

Directions:

- In a huge skillet, warm oil on medium heat.
- Put onion and sauté for approximately 4 minutes.
- Add garlic and jalapeño pepper and sauté for approximately 1 minute.
- Add beef and spices and cook approximately 6 minutes breaking into pieces while using spoon.
- Stir in tomatoes and greens and cook, stirring gently for about 4 minutes.
- Stir in lemon juice and take away from heat.

Nutrition:

Calories: 432

Fat: 16g

Carbohydrates: 27g

Fiber: 12g

Protein: 39g

Beef & Veggies Chili

Preparation Time: 15 minutes

Cooking Time: 1 hour

Servings: 6-8

Ingredients:

1. 2 pounds lean ground beef
2. ½ head cauliflower, chopped into large pieces
3. 1 onion, chopped
4. 6 garlic cloves, minced
5. 2 cups pumpkin puree
6. 1 teaspoon dried oregano, crushed
7. 1 teaspoon dried thyme, crushed
8. 1 teaspoon ground cumin
9. 1 teaspoon ground turmeric
10. 1-2 teaspoons chili powder
11. 1 teaspoon paprika
12. 1 teaspoon cayenne pepper
13. ¼ teaspoon red pepper flakes, crushed
14. Salt, to taste
15. Freshly ground black pepper, to taste
16. 1 (26 oz.) can tomatoes, drained
17. ½ cup water

18. 1 cup beef broth

Directions:

- Heat a substantial pan on medium-high heat.

- Add beef and stir fry for around 5 minutes.

- Add cauliflower, onion, and garlic and stir fry for approximately 5 minutes.

- Add spices and herbs and stir to mix well.

- Stir in remaining ingredients and provide to a boil.

- Reduce heat to low and simmer, covered approximately 30-45 minutes.

- Serve hot.

Nutrition:

Calories: 453

Fat: 10g

Carbohydrates: 20g

Fiber: 8g

Protein: 33g

Ground Beef & Veggies Curry

Preparation Time: 15 minutes

Cooking Time: 36 minutes

Servings: 6-8

Ingredients:

1. 2-3 tablespoons coconut oil
2. 1 cup onion, chopped
3. 1 garlic clove, minced
4. 1-pound lean ground beef
5. 1½ tablespoons curry powder
6. 1/8 teaspoon ground ginger
7. 1/8 teaspoon ground cinnamon
8. 1/8 teaspoon ground turmeric
9. Salt, to taste
10. 2½-3 cups tomatoes, chopped finely
11. 2½-3 cups fresh peas shelled
12. 2 sweet potatoes, peeled and chopped

Directions:

- In a sizable pan, melt coconut oil on medium heat.
- Add onion and garlic and sauté for around 4-5 minutes.

- Add beef and cook for about 4-5 minutes.
- Add curry powder and spices and cook for about 1 minute.
- Stir in tomatoes, peas, and sweet potato and bring to your gentle simmer.
- Simmer covered approximately 25 minutes.

Nutrition:

Calorie: 432

Fat: 16g

Carbohydrates: 21g

Fiber: 11g

Protein: 36g

Spicy & Creamy Ground Beef Curry

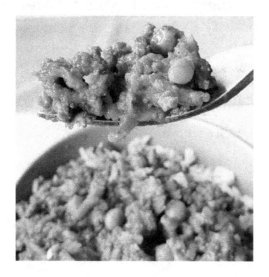

Preparation Time: 15 minutes

Cooking Time: 32 minutes

Servings: 4

Ingredients:

- 1-2 tablespoons coconut oil

- 1 teaspoon black mustard seeds

- 2 sprigs curry leaves

- 1 Serrano pepper, minced

- 1 large red onion, chopped finely

- 1 (1-inch) fresh ginger, minced

- 4 garlic cloves, minced

- 1 teaspoon ground coriander

- 1 teaspoon ground cumin

- ½ teaspoon ground turmeric

- ¼ teaspoon red chili powder

- Salt, to taste

- 1-pound lean ground beef

- 1 potato, peeled and chopped

- 3 medium carrots, peeled and chopped

- ¼ cup water

- 1 (14 oz.) can coconut milk

- Salt, to taste

- Freshly ground black pepper, to taste

- Chopped fresh cilantro, for garnishing

Directions:

1. In a big pan, melt coconut oil on medium heat.

2. Add mustard seeds and sauté for about thirty seconds.

3. Add curry leaves and Serrano pepper and sauté approximately half a minute.

4. Add onion, ginger, and garlic and sauté for about 4-5 minutes.

5. Add spices and cook for about 1 minute.

6. Add beef and cook for about 4-5 minutes.

7. Stir in potato, carrot, and water and provide with a gentle simmer.

8. Simmer, covered for around 5 minutes.

9. Stir in coconut milk and simmer for around fifteen minutes.

10. Stir in salt and black pepper and remove from heat.

11. Serve hot while using garnishing of cilantro.

Nutrition:

Calories: 432

Fat: 14g

Carbohydrates: 22g

Fiber: 8g

Protein: 39g

Curried Beef Meatballs

Preparation Time: 20 minutes

Cooking Time: 22 minutes

Servings: 6

Ingredients:

- For Meatballs:
- 1-pound lean ground beef
- 2 organic eggs, beaten
- 3 tablespoons red onion, minced
- ¼ cup fresh basil leaves, chopped
- 1 (1-inch fresh ginger piece, chopped finely
- 4 garlic cloves, chopped finely
- 3 Thai bird's eye chilies, minced
- 1 teaspoon coconut sugar
- 1 tablespoon red curry paste
- Salt, to taste
- 1 tablespoon fish sauce
- 2 tablespoons coconut oil
- For Curry:
- 1 red onion, chopped
- Salt, to taste

- 4 garlic cloves, minced

- 1 (1-inch) fresh ginger piece, minced

- 2 Thai bird's eye chilies, minced

- 2 tablespoons red curry paste

- 1 (14 oz.) coconut milk

- Salt, to taste

- Freshly ground black pepper, to taste

- Lime wedges, for

Directions:

1. For meatballs in a huge bowl, put all together the ingredients except oil and mix till well combined.

2. Make small balls from the mixture.

3. In a huge skillet, melt coconut oil on medium heat.

4. Add meatballs and cook for about 3-5 minutes or till golden brown all sides.

5. Transfer the meatballs right into a bowl.

6. In the same skillet, add onion and a pinch of salt and sauté for around 5 minutes.

7. Add garlic, ginger, and chilies, and sauté for about 1 minute.

8. Add curry paste and sauté for around 1 minute.

9. Add coconut milk and meatballs and convey to some gentle simmer.

10. Reduce the warmth to low and simmer, covered for around 10 minutes.

11. Serve using the topping of lime wedges.

Nutrition:

Calories: 444

Fat: 15g

Carbohydrates: 20g

Fiber: 2g

Protein: 37g

Beef Meatballs in Tomato Gravy

Preparation Time: 20 minutes

Cooking Time: 37 minutes

Servings: 4

Ingredients:

- For Meatballs:
- 1-pound lean ground beef
- 1 organic egg, beaten
- 1 tablespoon fresh ginger, minced
- 1 garlic oil, minced
- 2 tablespoons fresh cilantro, chopped finely
- 2 tablespoons tomato paste
- 1/3 cup almond meal
- 1 tablespoon ground cumin
- Pinch of ground cinnamon
- Salt, to taste
- Freshly ground black pepper, to taste
- ¼ cup coconut oil
- For Tomato Gravy:
- 2 tablespoons coconut oil
- ½ small onion, chopped

- 2 garlic cloves, chopped

- 1 teaspoon fresh lemon zest, grated finely

- 2 cups tomatoes, chopped finely

- Pinch of ground cinnamon

- 1 teaspoon red pepper flakes, crushed

- ¾ cup chicken broth

- Salt, to taste

- Freshly ground black pepper, to taste

- ¼ cup fresh parsley, chopped

Directions:

1. For meatballs in a sizable bowl, add all ingredients except oil and mix till well combined.

2. Make about 1-inch sized balls from the mixture.

3. In a substantial skillet, melt coconut oil on medium heat.

4. Add meatballs and cook for approximately 3-5 minutes or till golden brown all sides.

5. Transfer the meatballs into a bowl.

6. For gravy in a big pan, melt coconut oil on medium heat.

7. Add onion and garlic and sauté for approximately 4 minutes.

8. Add lemon zest and sauté approximately 1 minute.

9. Add tomatoes, cinnamon, red pepper flakes, and broth and simmer approximately 7 minutes.

10. Stir in salt, black pepper, and meatballs and reduce the warmth to medium-low.

11. Simmer for approximately twenty minutes.

12. Serve hot with all the garnishing of parsley.

Nutrition:

Calories: 404

Fat: 11g

Carbohydrates: 27g

Fiber: 4g

Protein: 38g

Pork with Lemongrass

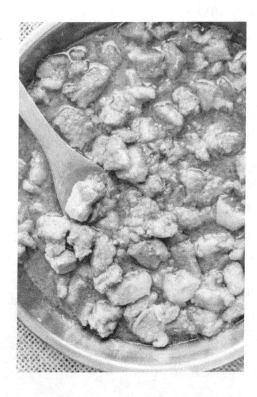

Preparation Time: 10 minutes

Cooking Time: 30 minutes

Servings: 4

Ingredients:

- 4 pork chops
- 2 tablespoons olive oil
- 2 spring onions, chopped
- A pinch of salt and black pepper

- ½ cup vegetable stock
- 1 stalk lemongrass, chopped
- 2 tablespoons coconut aminos
- 2 tablespoons cilantro, chopped

Directions:

1. Warm a pan with the oil on medium-high heat, add the spring onions, and the meat and brown for 5 minutes.
2. Add the rest of the ingredients, toss, and cook everything over medium heat for 25 minutes.
3. Divide the mix between plates and serve.

Nutrition:
Calories 290

Fat 4

Fiber 6

Carbs 8

Protein 14

Pork with Olives

Preparation Time: 10 minutes

Cooking Time: 40 minutes

Servings: 4

Ingredients:

- 1 yellow onion, chopped
- 4 pork chops
- 2 tablespoons olive oil
- 1 tablespoon sweet paprika
- 2 tablespoons balsamic vinegar
- ¼ cup kalamata olives, pitted and chopped
- 1 tablespoon cilantro, chopped
- Pinch of Sea Salt
- Pinch black pepper

Directions:

1. Warm a pan with the oil on medium heat; add the onion and sauté for 5 minutes.
2. Add the meat and brown for a further 5 minutes.
3. Put the rest of the ingredients, toss, cook over medium heat for 30 minutes, divide between plates and serve.

Nutrition:

Calories 280

Fat 11

Fiber 6

Carbs 10

Protein 21

Pork Chops with Tomato Salsa

Preparation Time: 10 minutes

Cooking Time: 15 minutes

Servings: 4

Ingredients:

- 4 pork chops
- 1 tablespoon olive oil
- 4 scallions, chopped
- 1 teaspoon cumin, ground
- ½ tablespoon hot paprika
- 1 teaspoon garlic powder
- Pinch of sea salt
- Pinch of black pepper
- 1 small red onion, chopped
- 2 tomatoes, cubed
- 2 tablespoons lime juice
- 1 jalapeno, chopped
- ¼ cup cilantro, chopped
- 1 tablespoon lime juice

Directions:

1. Warm a pan with the oil on medium heat, add the scallions and sauté for 5 minutes.
2. Add the meat, cumin paprika, garlic powder, salt, and pepper, toss, cook for 5 minutes on each side, and divide between plates.
3. In a bowl, combine the tomatoes with the remaining ingredients, toss, divide next to the pork chops and serve.

Nutrition:

Calories 313

Fat 23.7

Fiber 1.7

Carbs 5.9

Protein 19.2

Mustard Pork Mix

Preparation Time: 10 minutes

Cooking Time: 35 minutes

Servings: 4

Ingredients:

- 2 shallots, chopped
- 1 pound pork stew meat, cubed
- 2 garlic cloves, minced
- 2 tablespoons olive oil
- ¼ cup Dijon mustard
- 2 tablespoons chives, chopped
- 1 teaspoon cumin, ground
- 1 teaspoon rosemary, dried
- Pinch of sea salt
- Pinch black pepper

Directions:

1. Warm a pan with the oil on medium-high heat, add the shallots and sauté for 5 minutes.
2. Put the meat and brown for a further 5 minutes.
3. Put the rest of the ingredients, toss, and cook on medium heat for 25 minutes more.

4. Divide the mix between plates and serve.

Nutrition:

Calories 280

Fat 14.3

Fiber 6

Carbs 11.8

Protein 17

Pork with Chili Zucchinis and Tomatoes

Preparation Time: 10 minutes

Cooking Time: 35 minutes

Servings: 4

Ingredients:

- 2 tomatoes, cubed
- 2 pounds pork stew meat, cubed
- 4 scallions, chopped
- 2 tablespoons olive oil
- 1 zucchini, sliced
- Juice of 1 lime
- 2 tablespoons chili powder
- ½ tablespoons cumin powder
- Pinch of sea salt
- Pinch black pepper

Directions:

1. Warm a pan with the oil on medium heat, add the scallions and sauté for 5 minutes.
2. Add the meat and brown for 5 minutes more.

3. Add the tomatoes and the other ingredients, toss, cook over medium heat for 25 minutes more, divide between plates and serve.

Nutrition:

Calories 300

Fat 5

Fiber 2

Carbs 12

Protein 14

Pork with Thyme Sweet Potatoes

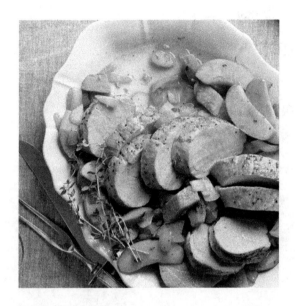

Preparation Time: 10 minutes

Cooking Time: 35 minutes

Servings: 4

Ingredients:

- 2 sweet potatoes, cut into wedges

- 4 pork chops

- 3 spring onions, chopped

- 1 tablespoon thyme, chopped

- 2 tablespoons olive oil

- 4 garlic cloves, minced

- Pinch of sea salt

- Pinch black pepper

- ½ cup vegetable stock

- ½ tablespoon chives, chopped

Directions:

1. In a roasting pan, combine the pork chops with the potatoes and the other ingredients, toss gently and cook at 390 degrees F for 35 minutes.

2. Divide everything between plates and serve.

Nutrition:
Calories 210

Fat 12.2

Fiber 5.2

Carbs 12

Protein 10

Pork with Pears and Ginger

Preparation Time: 10 minutes

Cooking Time: 35 minutes

Servings: 4

Ingredients:

- 2 green onions, chopped
- 2 tablespoons avocado oil
- 2 pounds pork roast, sliced
- ½ cup coconut aminos
- 1 tablespoon ginger, minced
- 2 pears, cored and cut into wedges
- ¼ cup vegetable stock
- 1 tablespoon chives, chopped

Directions:

1. Warm a pan with the oil on medium heat, add the onions, and the meat and brown for 2 minutes on each side.
2. Add the rest of the ingredients, toss gently, and bake at 390 degrees F for 30 minutes.
3. Divide the mix between plates and serve.

Nutrition:

Calories 220

Fat 13.3

 Fiber 2

Carbs 16.5

Protein 8

Parsley Pork and Artichokes

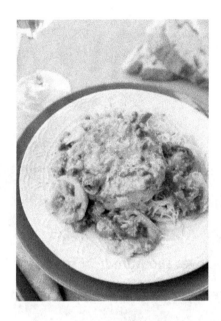

Preparation Time: 10 minutes

Cooking Time: 35 minutes

Servings: 4

Ingredients:

- 2 tbsp. balsamic vinegar
- 1 cup canned artichoke hearts, drained
- 2 tbsp. olive oil
- 2 lb. pork stew meat, cubed

- 2 tbsp. parsley, chopped

- 1 tsp. cumin, ground

- 1 tsp. turmeric powder

- 2 garlic cloves, minced

- Pinch of sea salt

- Pinch black pepper

Directions:

1. Warm a pan with the oil on medium heat, add the meat and brown for 5 minutes.

2. Add the artichokes, the vinegar, and the other ingredients, toss, cook over medium heat for 30 minutes, divide between plates and serve.

Nutrition:

Calories 260

Fat 5

Fiber 4

Carbs 11

Protein 20

Pork with Mushrooms and Cucumbers

Preparation Time: 10 minutes

Cooking Time: 25 minutes

Servings: 4

Ingredients:

- 2 tablespoons olive oil
- ½ teaspoon oregano, dried
- 4 pork chops
- 2 garlic cloves, minced
- Juice of 1 lime
- ¼ cup cilantro, chopped
- Pinch of sea salt
- Pinch black pepper
- 1 cup white mushrooms, halved
- 2 tablespoons balsamic vinegar

Directions:

1. Warm a pan with the oil on medium heat, add the pork chops and brown for 2 minutes on each side.

2. Put the rest of the ingredients, toss, cook on medium heat for 20 minutes, divide between plates and serve.

Nutrition:

Calories 220

Fat 6

Fiber 8

Carbs 14.2

Protein 20

Oregano Pork

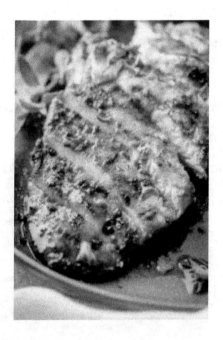

Preparation Time: 10 minutes

Cooking Time: 8 hours

Servings: 4

Ingredients:

- 2 pounds pork roast, sliced
- 2 tablespoons oregano, chopped
- ¼ cup balsamic vinegar
- 1 cup tomato paste
- 1 tablespoon sweet paprika

- 1 teaspoon onion powder

- 2 tablespoons chili powder

- 2 garlic cloves, minced

- A pinch of salt and black pepper

Directions:

1. In your slow cooker, combine the roast with the oregano, the vinegar, and the other ingredients, toss, put the lid on and cook on Low for 8 hours.

2. Divide everything between plates and serve.

Nutrition:
Calories 300

Fat 5

Fiber 2

Carbs 12,

Protein 24

Conclusion

The anti-inflammatory diet cookbook is the perfect resource for anyone who is suffering from inflammation. This cookbook has a special focus on reducing inflammation in the joints, cartilage, and muscles. Each recipe has been carefully developed to help reduce joint pain, joint stiffness, and even autoimmune disorders such as lupus and rheumatoid arthritis.

While most people associate food with comfort, a large number of foods are actually capable of having a dramatic impact on your health. Foods that are high in good fats (omega-3) are especially beneficial for many issues that affect the body. This cookbook provides recipes that are high in good fats and low in inflammatory foods like gluten and dairy. These recipes can be used to help create an anti-inflammatory diet that can help you feel better! The inflammatory disease will lead to many different health consequences and will even attack our most vital organs. The best way to do this is to prevent chronic inflammation in the first place. The next best thing is to recognize the signs and symptoms as early as possible, so proper interventions can be done to limit and reverse the impact of chronic inflammation. Inflammatory disease is the root cause of many long-term diseases, so ignoring the warning signs can create major consequences for your health.

Unfortunately, if the inflammatory disease gets out of control, preventative measures may be out of the question, and medical interventions will need to be done. Our goal is to prevent you from getting to this point. Lucky for us, many lifestyle changes can be performed to stop and reverse this disease process when it is still in its in advance stages. This is another reason why we should recognize and not ignore the signs and symptoms. A major lifestyle change we can commit to is a new diet plan. The anti-inflammatory diet is a meal plan that boasts healthy and nutritious cuisines, but still flavorful and appealing to the taste buds. There is a major myth out there that healthy food cannot be delicious. We have proven this myth wrong by providing numerous recipes from around the world that follow our healthy meal plan.

We hope that the information you read in this book gives you a better understanding of how the immune system functions and how a proper diet plan can help protect it and our other valuable cells and tissues. The recipes we have provided are just a starting point. Use them as a guide to create many of your dishes that follow the diet plan. Just make sure you use the proper ingredients and food groups. Also, for maximum results, follow the Anti-Inflammatory Diet food Guide Pyramid.

The next step is to take the instruction we have provided and begin taking steps to change your life and improve your health. Begin recognizing the signs and symptoms of chronic inflammation and make the necessary lifestyle changes to prevent further health problems. Start transitioning to the anti-inflammatory diet today by incorporating small meals into your schedule and increase the amount as tolerated. Within a short period, the diet will be a regular part of your routine. You will notice increased energy, improved mental function, a stronger and well-balanced immune system, reduction in chronic pain, some healthy weight loss, and overall better health outcomes. If you are ready to experience these changes, then wait no longer and begin putting your knowledge from this book into action.

CPSIA information can be obtained
at www.ICGtesting.com
Printed in the USA
BVHW090852260421
605871BV00002B/308